H

Apnea:

6th Edition

The Undeniable Truth on Which Therapies Actually

Work…

WITH 18 STRATEGIES TO BREATHE & SLEEP

EASY AGAIN

6TH EDITION INCLUDES BONUS BOOK:

Hacking CPAP Comfort — With 100+ CPAP Comfort

Hacks

Brady Nelson, RRT

Foreword by Sandeep Gill, RRT

Copyright © 2018 RespLabs Medical Inc.® All Rights Reserved.

No part of this publication may be reproduced, distributed, or transmitted in any form or by any means, including photocopying, recording, or other electronic or mechanical methods, or by any information storage and retrieval system without the prior written permission of the publisher, except in the case of very brief quotations embodied in critical reviews and certain other noncommercial uses permitted by copyright law.

For More Information, Visit: **RespLabs.com**

Foreword

Writing the foreword for this book was very special for me. I know Brady Nelson personally. He is easily the hardest working person I know.

Sleep apnea still is a common disease and very little is discussed about it. What is known is often confused with multiple treatment options. Most people do not know how it affects your health and it can lead to a cascade of diseases that are often treated symptomatically without treating the actual cause. The amount of information in our digital world is often confusing for most people. Some suggest CPAP, some suggest wearing oral devices, and some might deny the fact that their problem exists. (The latter being the least effective)

The average person sleeps about 8 hours a day, which is 1/3 of our entire life on average. We have to make sure we are getting good sleep so we can perform at our best. Every patient needs to discover the treatment that works best for him or her, and it's not always the choice they enjoy the most, initially. This is where this book becomes helpful; it helps patients find the option that best fits according to their needs.

Please enjoy.

Sandeep Gill, RRT

Why I Wrote This Book...

All you have to do is type the words "Sleep Apnea" in the kindle book search bar on Amazon.com. Seriously, try it. See for yourself.

As I am writing this, you will find a number of enticing titles. There's the "Sleep Apnea Cure Solution" and "The FREE Cure to Sleep Apnea, You Can Stop Using CPAP" ...

Sounds promising, doesn't it?

As a respiratory therapist, I've helped and treated thousands of patients. When I read the descriptions of these, I consider them extremely misleading.

Let's get a couple myths I've seen out of the way right now:

Essential oils are not a cure to sleep apnea. Neither is a ginger-carrot juice concoction. Neither is wearing an ionized copper bracelet.

There are even more blog posts online, doubling down on confusing everyone that there are FREE one-size-fits-all solutions or CUREs. As soon as we think we've seen them all, a new one pops up.

We've debunked some of the worst offenders here: https://www.youtube.com/watch?v=Ugyj5izMYQ4 (or Type in "Snoring Industry" or "Sleep Apnea Industry" on YouTube)

My goal is to give you an easy to understand explanation of what sleep apnea is. Then we will really dive into the treatment options available for patients and comment on what **ACTUALLY** works, from least invasive to most. Plus, now for existing CPAP users, we've added the bonus book Hacking CPAP Comfort, which is exclusive to our Updated 6th Edition.

If you, a friend, or a family member has recently been diagnosed with sleep apnea, or if you suspect you or someone you know has it, then this book is a great starting point. You don't need to read an 800-page book on sleep apnea to find out what will work best for you. That's why we've condensed everything you need to get the ball rolling.

This is now the 6th edition of this book, and we've had plenty of great feedback from readers, that have lead to updates in every chapter.

Some of this information will surprise and shock you.

I won't sugar coat anything. If there are even one or two points that you can take apply from this guide, we'll have succeeded.

Table of Contents:

Chapter 1: Sleep Apnea Explained

Cut to the Chase…

Sleep apnea or sleep-disordered breathing is simply when a person experiences one or more pauses in breathing during sleep. Each pause can last anywhere from a few seconds to a minute or more. These pauses can seriously reduce the oxygenation status of the body and lead to more jeopardizing conditions like a stroke or heart disease. Basically, the body needs a certain amount of oxygen to be maintained at all times. Pauses in breathing can jeopardize the amount of oxygen entering the body to the tissues and, of course, the brain.

Types of Sleep Apnea:

Obstructive Sleep Apnea –

This is, by far, the most common type of sleep apnea. The breathing pauses are caused by an obstruction in the airway. The obstruction most often occurs in the upper airway. The upper airway consists of the nasal cavities, soft palate, uvula, and the throat. Obstructions can occur at any point along the upper airway. Often when a person enters a deeper level of sleep, these soft tissues relax and can cause an obstruction to airflow. It is important to note that this type of sleep apnea is most often associated with snoring. However, just because someone snores, this does not mean they always have sleep apnea. (See figure 1 below: The base of the tongue is causing the obstruction in this patient) Note: We will also refer to positional sleep apnea in further chapters. This is a subset of patients with Obstructive Sleep Apnea.

Figure 1

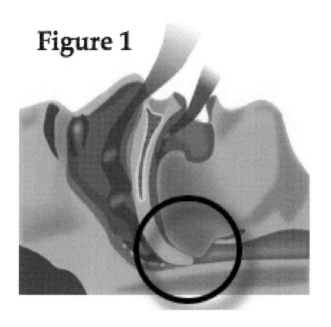

Credits to **Habib M'henni** / Wikimedia Commons

Central Sleep Apnea -

Central sleep apnea is a type of sleep apnea that is more difficult to treat and sometimes more dangerous then obstructive sleep apnea. The cause of the breathing pauses is from a misfire or delayed message from the central nervous system (brain and spinal cord). Either the brain fails to send the signal to the muscles that controls breathing, or the spinal cord fails to deliver the message.

This can be difficult to treat because the problem is with the brain and its signaling system.

Complex Sleep Apnea (or Mixed Sleep Apnea) –

This is a combination of obstructive sleep apnea and central sleep apnea.

Potential Complications

Sleep apnea can be brutal, not just for the person experiencing it, but also for the person trying to sleep next to them. If left untreated, sleep apnea can increase the risk for the following conditions:

- Heart attacks

- High blood pressure

- Diabetes

- Stroke

- Obesity

- Cardiac arrhythmias

- Accidents can occur at work or while driving because of poor concentration and fatigue.

In the next chapters, we are going to outline the different strategies to sleep and breathe easier. Please note that it is most important, before you act on any medical advice, that you consult your doctor. My goal here is to inform you, but everyone's situation is potentially very different.

Chapter 2: Getting to a Healthier Lifestyle

Go Figure...

Before we delve into the strategies, I want to make something really clear. Some of the strategies may not be as sexy and easy as you'd like them to be, and that's not what we're here for. Although you can find information on some of these treatments on the web, we're going to lay out which ones actually work and which ones don't, in the order of LEAST INVASIVE to MOST INVASIVE. Some strategies will work for one person and not another. Again, we reiterate how important it is to see your physician and get fully diagnosed, because everyone's case will be individual and different.

The forefront in improving sleep apnea is making healthier changes in lifestyle. Most often, people snore, and sleep apnea starts because of exposure to irritants such as cigarette smoke and other air pollutants causing inflammation. The condition can then worsen and may develop into a diagnosis of mild to severe sleep apnea. If the problem starts with poor health, then improvement would start by improving lifestyle and general health condition.

Strategy #1: Exercise & Diet

Improvement of any health condition always starts with making healthier choices. These include the following:

Eat well-balanced meals. This can help in achieving an ideal BMI and preventing excessive fat accumulation and weight that can put pressure on the airway and increase potential obstruction.

If you're looking for a current, and evidence-based diet resource, try searching Dr. William Davis. He is not only a cardiologist, but also behind the wheat belly diet if you've ever heard of it.

Exercise regularly to tone muscles. Yes, even if you just walk or jog for 30 minutes to an hour a day, this can help in improving sleep apnea. The point is that exercising can tone muscles that may increase the support of the airway. Note that the airway is composed of muscles and is surrounded by muscles. Even if the airway muscles are weak, the toned surrounding muscles can help support the airway and keep it from collapsing.

[1] A study from the ATS (American Thoracic Society) in 2009 speaks on losing weight as one of the most effective ways to cure sleep apnea. That being said, I also want to make really clear that in certain patients with sleep apnea, no amount of weight loss will help, even if you're at a healthy weight.

I Have a Question for You:

What big (or small) change can you make each day to improve your dietary choices and level of exercise?

What can you implement today? Like right now? Challenge yourself by setting a goal to improve your fitness level over the next 90 days. (Remember to never leave the sight of a goal without taking a small action towards achieving it.)

Strategy #2: Avoid Noxious Substances

Exposure to certain noxious substances can promote snoring, affect the strength and function of the airway, and promote the development of sleep apnea. By avoiding these substances, you can help in improving sleep apnea and snoring.

Quit smoking or start avoiding exposure to cigarette smoke. Several chemicals in cigarettes are noxious-irritating to the airway. The constant irritation can cause swelling and inflammation and create obstruction that can lead to sleep apnea.

[2] According to Lin YN (2012), "smoking cessation is recommended when considering treatment for OSA and treating OSA may be a necessary precondition for successful smoking cessation."

Avoid alcohol: Sorry, folks, but alcohol has a relaxing effect on the muscles. The relaxation can cause the airway or the tongue to fall back on each other and cause obstruction. Ever witnessed an intoxicated person asleep?

Notice how loud they snore. Sometimes they even snort in their sleep. Alcohol may help you go to sleep, but studies have shown that the quality of sleep is greatly reduced. Rapid eye movement (or REM sleep) is the "dreaming state" phase of sleep that our neurological system requires for learning. During this stage of sleep, rapid eye movements darting back and forth and up and down have been noted. Infants can spend up to 80% of their sleep cycles in REM state, whereas adults spend about 20%.

When alcohol is ingested before sleep, it was found by the London Sleep Centre in 2013 that [11] "the onset of the first REM sleep period is significantly delayed at all doses and appears to be the most recognizable effect of alcohol on REM sleep followed by the reduction in total night REM sleep."

Avoid sedatives: Just like alcohol, sedatives have a relaxing effect on the muscles. Avoid these to prevent the muscles of the airway from becoming too relaxed and collapsing.

I Have Another Question for You:

What big (or small) change can you make every day to decrease your exposure to noxious substances?

Is there anything you can implement today or tonight? Or right now? There is usually even a small change to make right away.

Chapter 3: Positional Therapy

Positional therapy is another treatment for snoring & sleep apnea.

This may work for people who experience sleep apnea episodes or snoring only while sleeping in the supine position (on their backs). This can often be referred to as positional sleep apnea. Usually it is due to the staple obstructive sleep apnea type, wherein the base of the tongue relaxes during sleep and falls on the back the throat. The tongue reduces the space through which air flow passes through the upper respiratory tract, often starting with snoring and then leading to apnea. For these patients, the solution is as simple as changing the way they sleep by sleeping on their sides.

During sleep, it is normal to toss and turn. Once one gets to sleep and rotates on one's back, snoring starts, and sleep apnea can occur. No one can be aware at all times not to sleep on their back.

There are therefore a few techniques that can help in preventing you from sleeping on your back, without having to wake up and constantly change positions...

Strategy #3: Positional Therapy

Is Positional Therapy Effective?

Many studies have been conducted to determine the effectiveness of therapy for positional sleep apnea. You will learn about other techniques that can also treat this in future chapters (such as CPAP or Mandibular Advancement Devices). Before we get to those, we'll discuss a few simpler methods that can work for specific populations.

One recent study conducted in 2012 [6] tested the long-term effect of positional therapy in patients with the positional type of OSA.

In this particular study, there were 16 participants. All of them were not able to tolerate the gold standard of OSA treatment, CPAP. They were given a positional therapy device. They performed a test night study first before they used the device. The positional therapy device was then used every night for the entire duration of the study — which lasted for 3 months. During the night, the participants were constantly monitored using an actigraphic recorder for objective measurement of OSA symptoms.

After the 3-month study, another follow-up study night was performed. The results from the first night (test night) were compared to the results from the follow-up study night. The conclusion was that positional therapy has the potential to effectively treat positional OSA.

Positional therapy only works for mild cases of OSA. Also, this only works if the obstruction is due to the upper airway or the tongue collapsing on the rest of the airways. Severe cases of sleep apnea will likely not respond to this kind of treatment. The airways will still collapse during sleep, regardless of the sleeping position assumed. Also, people suffering from central sleep apnea will not see any improvements in their condition with positional therapy.

Another point is that while this is a good option for those who cannot afford a sleep study, it is still better to have a study in order to determine if you have positional OSA.

Who Can Benefit from Positional Therapy?

CPAP remains the leading and most effective treatment for OSA. However, if CPAP is not well tolerated, people may try positional therapy techniques and find them helpful.

Devices Used for Positional Therapy

A very simple, cost-effective way of maintaining sleeping on your side is by using a tennis ball. The ball is placed inside a sock, and the sock is pinned to the back of the pajama top or shirt. When the person turns over on his or her back during sleep, the pressure from the ball is a source of discomfort, causing the person to immediately turn to the side again. This can occur without seriously disrupting sleep.

Aside from the tennis ball technique, there are products available on the market that work in much the same way. An example is the anti-snore shirt or a bumper belt. These devices keep the body in a sideways sleeping position by providing physical barriers that prevent one from turning over and sleeping on the back.

Other Techniques

If one tennis ball doesn't work, try sewing a pocket into the back of a pajama top or any shirt used for sleeping. Place 3 to 4 tennis balls inside this pocket. The uneven pressure from the balls will make the supine (lying on your back) position very uncomfortable, making the sideways position a better choice.

Fill a backpack with firm comfortable material, such as a flat, firm pillow. Wear this backpack during sleep. The extra bulk will make the supine position uncomfortable for sleep, causing you to assume the sideways position instead.

Keep in mind that these devices won't necessarily work for everyone, because not everyone has the exact same type of sleep apnea. Often times it's less to do with the devices and more to do with the severity of the patient's sleep apnea.

Chapter 4: The Chinstrap and Nasal Dilators

Strategy #4: Chinstraps

Chinstraps have two different uses. One is to keep the mouth closed to prevent airflow out of the mouth when using CPAP (More on CPAP in a later chapter). The other is to hold the jaw in a position (slightly forward) that keeps the upper airway open.

There was a study published in the Clinical Journal of Sleep Medicine in 2008 (Vorona RD, et al.) [7] suggesting that "A chinstrap alone improved severe obstructive sleep apnea as well as or better than the use of CPAP." Another article published in 2014 in the same journal by (Sushanth Bhat, M.D, et al) [8] suggested: "A chinstrap alone is not an effective treatment for OSA. It does not improve sleep disordered breathing, even in mild OSA, nor does it improve the AHI in REM sleep or supine sleep. It is also ineffective in improving snoring."

I want to make very clear that a chinstrap for keeping one's mouth closed using CPAP is very common and effective. What is not common or effective, in my experience and in the literature, is chinstraps used for treating sleep apnea on their own. Despite people buying them, I don't have much faith that these help with snoring much either.

A good example of this is if you look on Amazon.com and type in: Sleep Apnea Chin Straps. You'll notice that the reviews aren't that great for any of them. It's because people are being told they will cure snoring etc. The actual chinstrap products don't differ greatly, either.

A chinstrap in conjunction with specifically nasal CPAP or BiPAP therapy to prevent excessive oral air leaks is used with every kind of sleep apnea because you're treating specifically the air leak coming from the mouth.

If you do decide to try a chinstrap, here is some advice on optimizing it. Getting a comfortable fit may be a challenge. Try these tips to help get that good, comfortable chinstrap fit:

☐ Start by wearing the straps loose.

☐ Place the thumb ½ inch from the strip. Then, tear the strip and put it over the thumb.

☐ To avoid getting the hair caught in the straps, wrap a bit of cotton strip around the strap that will rest against the hair. Secure that strip of cotton by stitching it to the strap.

☐ Try the chinstrap back on and adjust to comfortable tightness. You should still be able to open your mouth while awake. The chinstrap is not to clamp the mouth tightly shut during sleep. Its main objective is to provide support for the jaw, keeping it in a closed, resting position. Clamping the mouth shut will only cause injury and undue strain on the muscles and bones of the jaw.

☐ The fit should be a gentle, secure hug over the head down to the chin. It shouldn't feel tight. The jaw should not feel tight and the teeth should not be grating together.

☐ Take the time to try different chinstrap positions to get the most comfortable one.

Strategy #5: Nasal Dilators

Nasal dilators are devices that attach to the nose to widen the opening of the nasal passages. Dilators can provide structural support to prevent collapse of the nasal tissues.

These may help for people who have a deviated nasal septum, which reduces the width of the nasal passages. However, the effectiveness of nasal dilators is very limited for sleep apnea. They may make it slightly easier to breathe, but they have little effect on sleep apnea and snoring, as these are more likely to take place due to the anatomy beyond the point at which the nasal dilators can provide support.

In other words, nasal dilators will only work for opening the nasal passages. They do not support the rest of the upper airway. They enhance the amount of airflow entering the nose, but don't necessarily affect the amount of air entering the rest of the airways. Nasal dilators will not work for those whose problems are from obstruction beyond the nasal passage.

A study published in CHEST (2000) by Schönhofer B. et al, [9] concluded: "The investigated nasal dilator had no effect on sleep-related breathing disorders in patients with moderate to severe OSA. The reduction in nasal resistance does not prevent hypopharyngeal obstruction."

There are many of these devices on the market. If you want to see what they look like, type in **Sleep Apnea Nasal Dilators** on Amazon.com.

This is another strategy that WILL work for a very SMALL population of sleep apnea patients, much like chinstraps alone. For $10-20 it might be worth a try, but in most sleep apnea patients, dilators won't help.

If you are going to try this, please note: the function of your nose is to heat, humidify & filter air & oxygen going into your lungs. Try to use a nasal dilator that doesn't entirely block nose hairs and the inside walls of your nose, so that your body can still do its job.

Chapter 5: Oral Appliance Therapy

Another treatment option for sleep apnea is the use of various types of oral appliances. Oral appliance therapy involves wearing a removable oral appliance inside the mouth during sleep. Most appliances resemble an orthodontic retainer, or a mouth guard used in sports.

Is It Effective?

The oral appliance is gaining some traction and becoming a treatment plan. It is an effective first line of treatment for some people suffering from sleep apnea. The AASM has also approved these as a first-line treatment plan for people who suffer from mild to moderate types of sleep apnea. This is also recommended for those with severe sleep apnea who cannot tolerate CPAP. Sometimes, oral appliances are used together with a CPAP in order to provide both benefits.

What Are Oral Appliances for and How Do They Work?

The main goal of the oral appliance is to prevent the airways from collapsing by supporting the lower jaw and holding the tongue forward. This way, the oral appliance prevents the tongue from collapsing down into the throat to cause an obstruction. Also, by keeping the jaw forward, the muscles in the upper airway are pulled up to prevent collapsing down and causing an obstruction.

The oral appliance must be custom fitted in order to be effective. Each individual's oral cavity is different in terms of dimensions and needs. Hence, no two appliances are ever exactly the same. Purchase one that is solely and purposefully made according to your fit. There are also over-the-counter oral appliances available, but these are highly discouraged to for use in treating snoring or OSA.

The below figure is an example of an oral appliance used to treat OSA.

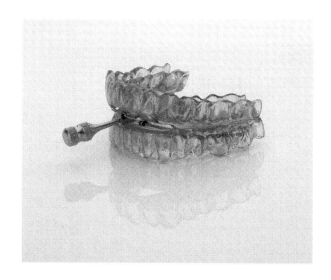

Figure 2.0 https://commons.wikimedia.org/wiki
File%3AOrthoapnea_%2C_oral_appliance.jpg

Strategy #6: Mandibular Advancement Devices

These are appliances that reposition the patient's lower jaw, putting it in a more forward and slightly downward position. This position helps to keep the airways open during sleep. This type is the most widely used type of oral appliance for the treatment of sleep apnea.

Something I want to make you aware of is that if you were to search somewhere like Amazon or many places online (on Amazon, type in Mandibular Advancement Device), you'll find a variety of devices. Most of these devices, considered "boil-and-bites," will potentially support the lower jaw in place, but will not advance the lower jaw. To advance the lower jaw, you typically need to receive a device that is custom made for you by a dentist who specializes in sleep medicine. Oral appliance therapy may seem like an exciting treatment because of its ease of use, but it is still not the leading treatment. The side effects are few, but some users may experience:

☐   Excessive salivation

- [ ] Temporary changes in bite
- [ ] Discomfort (minor) in the jaw and teeth

There are also a few potential complications in some users, which include:

- [ ] TMJ symptoms
- [ ] Permanent bite changes
- [ ] Lower jaw pain

Only a week ago (when this section was written) I ran into an old acquaintance that I'd met through a sleep apnea awareness project we did almost 8 years ago and hadn't seen each other since then. Interestingly enough, his father is a very accomplished dentist, and the creator of one of the first & most successful oral appliances for sleep apnea on the market.

They also have a great over the counter oral appliance (probably one of the best) that they were marketing heavily a few years ago. The problem was, and still is, that very severe sleep apnea patients would turn to this device. However, oral appliances are truly made and recommended for milder to moderate levels of severity. Hence, much of the time, these patients failed on them; because they weren't suitable for it in the first place.

Strategy #7: Boil-and-Bites

As mentioned, pre-made, ready-to-use oral appliances for sleep apnea are available at drugstores and online. These are very often not FDA-approved and may have risks associated with them.

Some people choose these "boil-and-bites" because, by choosing this option, they do not have to undergo a series of diagnostic tests and custom fittings. These boil-and-bites are named so because you buy them, boil them to sanitize and soften them, and then bite into them while they are soft. This makes for a decent fit once they harden again.

Another attraction of these ready-made oral appliances is that people do not have to wait for their fitted oral appliance before they can use them and experience relief. However, the oral cavity is unique in each person. These pre-made oral appliances may not always be a perfect fit. This can cause side effects that can turn into serious complications. Poorly fitting oral appliances can cause tooth movement (false dentures are less desirable than having to wait for a custom-made oral appliance) and jaw problems (e.g., TMJ problems, which are more painful and more of a hassle to treat than sleep apnea with an oral appliance). At times, sleep apnea can worsen when using poorly fitting oral appliance.

How Do I Get a Custom-Made Oral Appliance?

Custom-made oral appliances are fitted and made by dentists trained for treatment of sleep apnea. These trained dental professionals conduct a full evaluation of the TMJ (temporomandibular joint), mouth, and teeth. Part of the evaluation is to make sure that the jaw and the teeth are healthy and strong enough for an oral appliance. Loose teeth, swollen or infected gums, and jaw instability are some of the contraindications to wearing an oral appliance, because the appliance can cause more problems. After an evaluation and measurements are made, models of the patient's teeth will be made. Then a follow-up appointment is scheduled. In the next visit, the custom oral appliance will be fitted to the patient.

The custom-made oral appliance is adjustable. Your dentist will work with you to monitor progress and to keep your jaw perfectly and properly aligned. Regular dental appointments with a trained dentist for sleep apnea are required to check for response to the appliance in terms of improvement in OSA. These appointments also aim to check for both fit and effectiveness.

Strategy #8: Tongue Retaining Devices

Tongue retaining devices are designed and used to hold the tongue in place during sleep. By holding the tongue in place, these oral appliances keep the airway open, preventing apnea. Type "Tongue Retaining Device" on Amazon for an example.

The success of these devices is summarized well in a study published in the Journal of Clinical Sleep Medicine in 2009 by [10] Diane S. Lazard, M.D, et al:

"Tongue-retaining device performance tended to be similar to that of the mandibular advancement device. Thus, teams trained in tongue-retaining device fabrication and fitting may propose it as an alternative to continuous positive airway pressure, taking nasal obstruction into consideration as a contraindication."

Furthermore, it is best to have a tongue-retaining device fitted and manufactured by a professional if your diagnosis proves that this may be a viable option.

Chapter 6: Positive Airway Pressure Devices

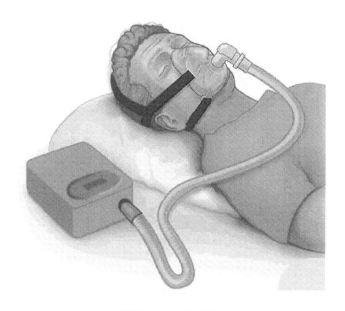

By PruebasBMA (Own work) [CC BY-SA 3.0
(http://creativecommons.org/licenses/by-sa/3.0)], via Wikimedia Commons

Positive Airway Pressure devices are the machines you may have seen before that come with various types of masks. They are widely used in the treatment of mild to severe sleep apnea. The American Academy of Sleep Medicine (AASM) endorses them as the most effective treatment.

Basically, Positive Airway Pressure machines work by placing the mask over the patient's nose, or nose and mouth, depending on the patient's needs. The mask should be worn snugly during sleep. Pressurized air is then delivered continuously through the mask and into the person's lungs. The increase in air pressure continuously passing through the airway tract keeps the airways open to prevent collapse at all angles of anatomy (something that an oral appliance or positional therapies will not achieve).

A flexible tube carries the pressurized air into the mask. The air is generated (or pressurized) within the machine. There are several types of machines for this. These include:

- Continuous Positive Airway Pressure (**CPAP**)

- Bi-level Positive Airway Pressure (**BiPAP or BPAP**)

- Variable Positive Airway Pressure (**VPAP or ASV**)

Results of thousands of studies have consistently shown that these machines do help alleviate sleep apnea.

Strategy #9: CPAP

Continuous Positive Airway Pressure (CPAP) is the most popular and most widely used type of Positive Airway Pressure devices. It is also the most common treatment used for mild, moderate and severe types of sleep apnea. It works by supplying a steady stream of air at one pressure level. With the continuous airflow, pressure is exerted against the airways. This is what keeps the airways open and prevents the collapse that causes sleep apnea.

A respiratory therapist, polysomnographic technologist, or a sleep doctor determines the amount of air pressure needed. The amount of pressure should fit the needs of the individual and depends solely on the amount of pressure needed to keep the airway open during sleep. A CPAP titration study may be recommended in order to calibrate the individual's air pressure setting.

The CPAP device and masks are continuously evolving and becoming more comfortable for patients. Most often the masks range from a full-face to nasal mask. There are other options, ranging from a total facemask to nasal prong style. The goal is to fit each individual patient's needs.

If I haven't emphasized it enough above, I will now: CPAP and other positive pressure devices will work for most people with sleep apnea and the hard FACT is, they save lives. The biggest problem is giving up on it too early and not being set-up or properly fitted in the first place. For some people, it is really easy to get used to, while others, it can be challenging, but incredibly worth it. For someone's first hand story, from a great writer, see Phil Elmore's book listed at the end of this.

Tips for Using CPAP (and some troubleshooting tips):

It will take some time to get used to the CPAP device. It is normal to feel uncomfortable at first. To make the experience more comfortable, try these tips:

☐ **Perfect Fit:** Most discomfort is due to a misfit. The correct fit of the mask will make a huge difference in terms of comfort and results. The strap of the mask should not be too loose or too tight. The mask should be large enough to completely seal over the nose and/or the mouth. The mask should have a good seal in order to maintain the right airway pressure and continuous airflow. Make a regular appointment to check that the mask still fits great. The straps can loosen over time, so it is best to check for fit regularly. Also, go for regular treatment evaluations to make sure that the settings and the entire treatment plan are working and appropriate. Again, CPAP is a great treatment option for obstructive sleep apnea, but individual responses may differ.

- **Easing into the CPAP:** Start slowly. Use the CPAP for short periods at first, preferably during the day. This will give you time to get used to the device. Using the CPAP for the first time at night can lead to too much discomfort and may add to sleep disturbance. Also, set the device to the "ramp" setting, which is available on most devices. When the ramp is set by a healthcare professional, it is used to gradually increase the air pressure when the CPAP is first turned on, allowing you time to get accustomed to the airflow. Some people may take a few weeks to months to get used to it.

- **Consider Customizing:** CPAP masks are available in various sizes. To get that perfect fit, you may need to continue to customize. Have the tube, straps and especially the mask customized to achieve the best fit and to get the right setup. Also, the availability of soft pads may help reduce skin irritation or strap marks. Also, consider discussing with your doctor the use of a nasal pillow style mask to reduce nasal discomfort. For a list of resources, visit: HackingSleepApnea.com.

☐ **Use Your Humidifier:** Most modern positive airway pressure devices come with an attached heated humidifier. This can help in reducing dryness in the airway, which is something that can commonly occur without the use of a humidifier. With standard humidifier containers, it is best practice to use distilled or deionized water. You can get distilled water just about anywhere. Heated tubing may also add to your comfort while using the CPAP machine. As water cools, it produces water droplets (condensate) and this can get into your mask and slosh back and forth in your tubing when you are sleeping. Adding a heated tubing system to your humidified CPAP machine may help this problem.

☐ **Get a CPAP Pillow:** Here I find some people find that these don't help at all, and some people absolutely love theirs, have more than one, and will never sleep without it. There are several different styles, but typically they have custom cut-outs for each side that prevents mask movement when sleeping on your side, reducing the chance of mask leaks. For a recommended pillow, visit HackingSleepApnea.com

☐ **CPAP Aromatherapy:** There are essential oil brands and products used specially for CPAP devices. Before you go shopping for any of these, please know this: **Do Not** place any type of these products directly in your humidifier. I've heard many people ask this. None of these products are made for that and can potentially make you very sick. The correct way to use them is to set up a device (such as a piece of cotton on a stand with some oil and adequate space) behind the air intake of the machine.

☐ **CPAP Moisturizer:** There are specific products to relieve dry nose and lips used for this that are customized petroleum free. This is considered important in patients that specifically require higher oxygen concentrations through their CPAP devices. Regular moisturizers may not be suitable to your mask material as well. For a recommended product visit HackingSleepApnea.com

☐ **Keep the Device Clean**: Make sure that the CPAP machine, the mask, straps, headgear, and the tubes are always clean. Clean and dry after each use to discourage bacterial, fungal, or mold growth. CPAP Mask Wipes can be used to clean daily. Once a week it is advised to use a baby shampoo and water to do a thorough clean. Replacing CPAP filters every 4 weeks is recommended. There are CPAP tubing cleaners that will help with cleaning the inside of the tubing as well. It is recommended to replace CPAP tubing once a year. Cleanliness of the entire device and all its attachments will aide in getting maximum benefit and comfort. This also reduces the risk of infection from microbial growth in dirty devices. If you are interested in automating the cleaning and sanitizing process, there are relatively small standalone units you can get for your home for a price. For a list of recommended products, visit HackingSleepApnea.com.

Strategy #10 Bi-Level Positive Airway Pressure

Bi-level Positive Airway Pressure (BiPAP) devices are used as an alternative to CPAP. Often, higher-pressure levels are achieved with BiPAP. It is most often used when CPAP isn't enough to effectively treat a patient's apnea. This mode is also used with patient's suffering from central sleep apnea that have weak breathing patterns.

This device adjusts air pressure between two different pressure levels during sleep. It provides more pressure during inhalation and then reduces the pressure upon exhalation. Some devices have a detection unit, which is set to deliver a breath automatically when it detects that the person has not taken one within a certain number of seconds. This is especially helpful in central sleep apnea.

ASV (adaptive servo-ventilation) devices are designed to help those suffering from both central and obstructive sleep apnea. The term "adaptive" refers to the device's capability to adjust its settings according to the patient's normal breathing patterns. The device automatically adjusts and delivers airflow pressure needed to prevent apnea or pauses in breathing while the person is asleep.

Chapter 7: Stimulation Therapy

The FDA recently approved a new treatment option for sleep apnea. This is called stimulation therapy or, more accurately, upper airway stimulation therapy.

Strategy #11 Upper Airway Stimulation Therapy

What is Upper Airway Stimulation Therapy?

This sleep apnea treatment plan uses a small device implanted into the patient. This device will sense the patient's breathing patterns. Then, it will mildly stimulate the key airway muscles to keep the airways open during sleep. There are no tubes, oral appliances or masks required for this. However, there are 3 components of the stimulator, which are all fully implanted. There is a small generator, a stimulation lead, and a breathing sensor.

The implantation procedure is done on an outpatient basis. The procedure generally lasts for two hours or less while the patient is under general anesthesia. After the anesthesia wears off and the patient is stable, they can go home that same day.

Once home, the device is only turned on before going to bed. Then, when getting up in the morning, the patient turns the device off. The on-off switch is a hand-held sleep remote. Using this device is easy and very simple. Those who have it don't have to worry about frequent setting adjustments each night, nor do they have to deal with tubes, appliances, masks, and other equipment.

Who are Candidates for Upper Airway Stimulation Therapy?

People can qualify for this type sleep apnea treatment if they meet these conditions:

- ☐ Diagnosed with obstructive sleep apnea (OSA)

- ☐ Did not tolerate, or condition failed to improve with, CPAP therapy

☐ No other implantable devices currently in use, such as a pacemaker

☐ No conditions or diseases that may otherwise disqualify a person for the procedure, such as blood clots (or clotting problems) and current sepsis or other infection

If a patient meets the above criteria, a sleep assessment will be performed under the supervision of a sleep medicine specialist. This is to evaluate the type of sleep apnea and its severity.

The patient may possibly also need an endoscopy in order to determine which anatomy is causing the sleep apnea. An endoscopy is inserting a tube fitted with a tiny camera into the airways while the patient is under sedation. This is done to examine which part of the airway is causing the obstruction. After all these assessment procedures are conducted, the sleep doctor will then make a recommendation as to whether upper airway stimulation therapy is indicated.

What to Expect After the Implant Procedure?

After the stimulation device is implanted, expect that there will be a small amount of pain and swelling at the site of incision. This can last for a few days. However, the pain and swelling should gradually go down in the next few days. If it worsens, have the incision site checked immediately. Also, pain and swelling should not interfere with normal, non-strenuous, daily activities. Full recovery is expected within two weeks.

A week after the implant procedure, the patient will return to the doctor to have the site examined. The incision will be evaluated for proper healing and absence of infection or other potential complications. About three to four weeks after the procedure, another appointment will be made. In this second appointment, the device will be turned on for the first time and then set by the sleep physician.

After a few months of use, another follow-up appointment is made. During this appointment, the sleep physician will conduct an overnight sleep study. This will evaluate the device's effectiveness and check if the patient is responding well to the treatment plan. Also, the settings of the device will be re-adjusted to suit the patient's needs, if indicated.

Aside from these appointments, general check-ups are also advised once or twice a year while having the stimulation device.

The device's battery generally lasts for 10 years. Battery replacements are done through an outpatient procedure.

Is This Effective?

This treatment plan is most recommended for people suffering from moderate to severe types of sleep apnea who cannot use, tolerate, or improve with CPAP therapy. This is also an alternative option for those who are candidates for surgery but who do not want to consider further surgical procedures for their sleep apnea.

This treatment option is not for everyone. CPAP still remains the gold standard for sleep apnea. But this is effective for people who are struggling with CPAP use and those who want to try alternative treatment options.

Several studies have already been conducted to determine the effectiveness of upper airway stimulation therapy. One notable recent study by Soose RJ, et al, [11] involved 126 participants. About 83% of the participants were men. The participants were recruited from 22 different sites across the US. The participants were carefully chosen, based on particular criteria — being unable to tolerate positive airway pressure. Other criteria considered for the selection of participants included a diagnosis of a moderate to severe case of sleep apnea, apnea episodes that were moderate to moderately severe, and exhibitions that the cause of sleep apnea was due to an obstruction at the level of the tongue.

In this study, two parameters were used to determine the treatment's efficacy. One was through an apnea-hypopnea index. This is a measurement of how many apnea events occur in 1 hour. The other parameter calculated is the oxygen desaturation index. This refers to how many times the level of oxygen in the blood falls by more than 4% in one hour of sleep.

The participants underwent 12 months of stimulation therapy. At the end of the study period, participants showed a 68% decrease in their scores for the apnea-hypopnea index. They also exhibited a 70% increase in their scores for the oxygen desaturation index.

After the 12-month study, the researchers further made a sub-study. Of the participants, 23 people continued with the stimulation therapy for one week. Another 23 participants were retained in the sub-study but did not continue with the treatment. Their apnea-hypopnea index scores were compared. Results showed that the participants who stopped their treatment for a week had higher apnea-hypopnea index scores. They also experienced more snoring and were more fatigued during the day. Those who continued with the treatment retained their improvements.

Some of the participants did report some pain and discomfort over the incision site. This is common and expected after any surgical procedure, even something minor like implanting a device. The pain level is also much, much less than the pain after undergoing a surgical procedure involving the upper airways.

Also, researchers did not find any prolonged issues concerning the tongue. After implantation, a few participants did report some weakness in the tongue, but the concern quickly faded after some time.

This is probably one of the most exciting alternative treatments in a long time. However, I tried to outline the entire procedure so that you can see it is more invasive than working with CPAP or any other treatments spoken about prior to this point. If you're interested in learning more, Inspire Sleep is one of the companies right now that has this type of product on the market.

Chapter 8: Surgery

In some patients, surgery might be an option as a treatment for sleep apnea. People who cannot tolerate CPAP or who are not responding to CPAP therapy are likely candidates. This is the most invasive treatment plan and is often reserved as the last resort.

Surgery is performed to increase the diameter of the airways to reduce sleep apnea episodes. The surgical procedures may involve the removal of excess tissue inside the nose or at the back of the throat (if present and causing OSA), the adenoids, or the tonsils. Surgery may also have to involve reconstruction of the jaw to widen the upper airways.

Is it Effective?

Surgery can help those who have exhausted other treatment options but who still suffer from sleep apnea. However, in some cases the risks of surgery may outweigh the benefits.

Surgery comes with its own risks. For some people, their sleep apnea symptoms and episodes even become worse after they undergo surgery. Then, too, there are the usual risks that come with any surgery, such as post surgical infection, high levels of pain at the surgical site, a few days of having to endure limited activities and limited movement, a worsening of apnea symptoms, and unforeseen injuries to the surgical site. All these may create more serious problems. Other negative aspects of undergoing surgery include:

- Swelling and bleeding in the throat

- The jaw is wired shut (if the surgery involves manipulating or reconstructing the jaws) for days

- Limited diet while the surgical site heals

- Hospital stay

Some surgeries for sleep apnea are minimally invasive. Some can be complex. The ultimate goal of surgery is to treat the involved area. It may involve repositioning, stiffening, or removing tissues of the throat.

Also, surgery is not a one-time, cure-all method. There are so many potential sites of obstruction. Finding out exactly what site or sites are to be surgically fixed is not as easy as performing a conventional sleep study or a single diagnostic effort. It takes a team to determine what areas are contributing to the problem. Also, it may take more than a single surgery to fix everything.

Strategy #12: LAUP

Laser-Assisted Uvuloplasty (LAUP): With this procedure, the surgeon makes several cuts on the soft palate with a laser. These cuts are allowed to form scar tissue. The scar formation will tighten the tissues of the soft palate. On the next several visits, the uvula is gradually trimmed. This procedure is considerably less painful compared to the UPPP you'll learn about next. This also has fewer side effects. However, the effectiveness is also comparable to UPPP.

Strategy #13: UPPP

Uvulopalatopharyngoplasty (UPPP): This is one of several surgeries involving the soft palate located at the roof of the mouth, towards the back portion of the throat. UPPP removes and repositions the excess tissues in the throat in order to widen the airway. The uvula and the soft palate are also trimmed, the tonsils are removed, and some of the soft palate muscles repositioned. The effectiveness of this procedure is variable. The UPPP procedure is not enough to treat moderate to severe cases of sleep apnea. Some patients report being worse off after having the procedure.

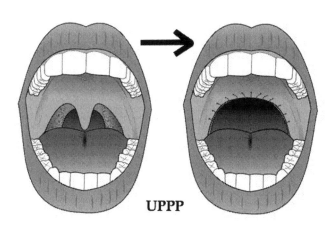

UPPP

By Drcamachoent (Own work) [CC BY-SA 4.0
(http://creativecommons.org/licenses/by-sa/4.0)], via Wikimedia Commons

Strategy #14 Septoplasty & Turbinate Reduction

This is a kind of nasal surgery. The main goal of septoplasty is to straighten a deviated or bent nasal septum, improving the size of the opening of the nasal passages. Turbinate reduction is a procedure that removes or reduces the curved structure sticking from the sides of the nose. This surgery will not be effective if the sleep apnea is caused by anatomy past the nasal anatomy.

Strategy #15: Palatal Implants

This procedure can be effective in reducing snoring and improving episodes of mild sleep apnea. Small rods made of fiberglass are inserted into the patient's soft palate. The goal of the fiber rods is to provide structural support to stiffen and strengthen the soft palate tissue and prevent blockage of the airway.

Strategy #16: MMO and MMA

Maxillomandibular Osteotomy and Advancement:

This is a surgical option for severe cases of sleep apnea. The upper and/or the lower jaws are moved forward in order to enlarge the breathing space within the throat. This procedure includes cutting the bones of the jaw to make the needed adjustments. Healing takes months. The jaw will have to be wired shut for approximately a week. Diet is also limited to liquids for this period of time.

Strategy #17: Weight Loss Surgeries

Obesity has a huge impact on sleep apnea. The excess weight the body carries can put undue strain or pressure on the upper airways. The excess fat may also press on the throat structures, constricting them and causing obstruction.

One type of weight loss surgery is bariatric surgery. This can promote weight loss in people suffering from severe obesity and sleep apnea. While this does help improve episodes of sleep apnea, it is recommended more to reduce the complications of obesity rather than for sleep apnea.

Strategy #18 — Tracheostomy

Over the years, I have worked with patients in the hospital with this procedure, but most often it is not used for sleep apnea.

Tracheostomy tube insertion is an effective surgical procedure for sleep apnea but is also among the most invasive and drastic options. This is reserved for rare emergency situations. However, tracheostomies are actually not all that rare, just rare for sleep apnea patients.

This procedure involves making a small hole in the trachea and then inserting a tube directly into the patient's windpipe. The tube can be capped during the day, so the person can breathe and talk normally. At night, before going to sleep, the cap is removed and therefore, the tube is opened to allow breathing., The tracheostomy tube functions as a secondary airway to the upper airway (where the obstruction may be severe).

Please also note that in severe cases of central sleep apnea, (especially in children), a tracheostomy tube may be indicated to facilitate nocturnal ventilation. In this case, the tracheostomy tube would be plugged during the day as tolerated so the person can breathe and speak. At nighttime, the tracheostomy tube would be unplugged, and the person would be attached to a ventilator to facilitate breathing,

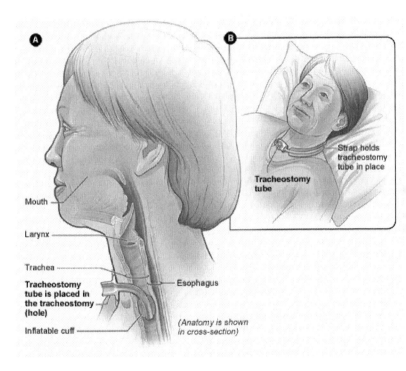

By National Heart Lung and Blood Institute (NIH) (National Heart Lung and Blood
Institute (NIH)) [Public domain], via Wikimedia Commons

Commentary on Provent, Airing, & Metamason:

I haven't added these to the strategies yet, for a few reasons that you'll see below:

Provent:

If you're not familiar with Provent, it is a circular adhesive, slightly larger than a nostril. Each adhesive has a one-way valve to allow airflow into the nose, then restrict airflow out of the nose on exhalation. This creates backpressure that keeps the upper-airway open to prevent obstructive apnea. Provent is approved by the FDA. There is media online that state it is an alternative for CPAP in mild, moderate, & severe sleep apnea patients. I don't particularly agree with this, especially when it comes to severe cases of sleep apnea.

As we discussed earlier, there are alternatives to CPAP, and for a small population perhaps this may help. I don't want to discredit this company's work and would love to learn more from them. But for most sleep apnea patients, the problem exists on inspiration. A device in this category MIGHT help on exhalation, likely in very mild cases at best.

Airing:

This is probably the most exciting news to hit the sleep apnea market in years. For those that haven't heard of it, you can check it out on YouTube. Sleep clinics across the country get calls from patients about this new technology daily. Patients wonder when it will be available, and doctors want it for their patients.

I'll give you a bit more background if you haven't heard of it. Airing is a small device that sits just under your nose and fits snugly, just like a nasal pillow mask, into each nostril. It requires very minimal space, is battery operated, and requires no CPAP tubing.

The company raised a million dollars in a crowd-funding campaign to try to get this product to market. I apologize if I am bursting any bubbles. My thoughts on this are that we are a VERY LONG way away from having an effective sleep apnea treatment in a device this size. I'd really like to be proven wrong, because this would change the landscape of sleep apnea therapy. I love thoughtful/innovative technology. It is incredibly exciting, but I wouldn't get anyone's hopes up that this will be available on the market soon.

Metamason:

This is one technology that seems very close, which you can be more excited about. Metamason is a 3D printing and scanning technology that can build truly customized masks for CPAP/BiPAP patients.

As you are now aware, one of the biggest hurdles in fitting CPAP masks with any patient is the one-size-fits-all choices available. Don't get me wrong; there are a lot of sizes and types of masks available, and most patients will be good. But to have a truly customized fit for your independent facial features would make a massive difference in the time and labor it takes fitting a patient correctly. My guess is that it will be at a premium, but for many people, probably well worth it. It seems they will be starting with nasal pillow type masks once FDA approved.

Quick Notes from The Field:

These are just a few notes that come to mind that can hopefully leave you with a few more tips. Some, we already talked about, but I will expand on them here.

1. What are people referring to AHI for? AHI is an acronym for Apnea-Hypopnea Index. It is the most common indicator of sleep apnea severity. It is measured as the number of events (apneas or hypopneas) that occur during an hour of sleep. A normal person may have between 0-4. A mild case of sleep apnea is between 5-14 events. A moderate case is between 15-29, and severe is greater than 30 events in an hour. Some institutions also use what is called the DI or desaturation index.

2. When getting used to a CPAP machine, take advantage of the ramp feature that is on most machines. This will make it easier to for you to get used to the device by starting the machine off at a lower pressure. Over 10 minutes or more, the machine will slowly "ramp" up to the needed pressure to maintain an open airway.

3. One of the most common reasons for nasal congestion is an improperly set humidifier. Make sure the humidifier is turned on at the most reasonable and tolerable heat level. The higher the heat, the more humidity will be carried in the air.

4. Can you use tap water in a humidifier? In most cases, if the water is treated carefully, it probably won't hurt. It is recommended to use distilled water, though, because the minerals in tap water will leave sediment in the humidifier. If the tap water is untreated, it can be a source of infection, which is carried into the lungs.

5. **One Last Thing**. I've seen many "magic juice recipes" and other totally misleading articles online saying they'll cure sleep apnea. You obviously know now that sleep apnea is a little more complex than a special ginger carrot juice recipe can fix. All in all, just be wary of any new exciting treatment options that seem too good to be true.

Pediatric & Infant Sleep Apnea

Several times now we've had email feedback saying to include information about sleep apnea in kids in this book. My wife Alisha is a registered respiratory therapist at BC Children's Hospital in Vancouver and manages the at home ventilation and tracheostomy program. Below is from her as I feel she is more qualified to comment on this:

Yes- you read that title right. Infants and children can have symptoms of obstructive or even central sleep apnea. Actually, anatomically children are at a disadvantage compared to adults. Children have a small jaw in relation to their tongue size which can make it easier for them to obstruct at night. They also have larger head in relation to the rest of their anatomy. This makes them [12] "obligatory nasal breathers" and if they are sick with a cold, they are at an increased risk of respiratory compromise.

Children are diagnosed and prescribed positive airway pressure for many different reasons. Some may include:

1. Pierre Robin Sequence

2. Micrognathia

3. Large tonsils and adenoids

4. Down Syndrome

5. Cerebral Palsy

6. Childhood obesity

7. Anatomical Variant

Symptoms of sleep apnea in children are similar to those in adults. Some may include morning headaches, difficulty staying awake during the day, behavioral issues, difficulty concentrating and witnessed snoring or obstructive episodes by family members.

If you suspect your child has sleep apnea, it is best to bring it up with your child's doctor. Your doctor will then likely refer you to a pediatric respirologist for further testing. If it is determined that your child has sleep apnea either through an overnight pulse oximetry test or polysomnography test, the respirologist will determine which treatment best suits your child's individual case.

The good news is, the non-invasive positive airway pressure devices and masks that provide both CPAP and Bi-Level ventilation have greatly improved overtime. These innovative machines have made it easier to apply this therapy to children as young as new born babies!

Some Tips on Getting Your Child Used to CPAP

Try getting them to wear it during the day when they are watching their favorite show. They are likely to be distracted by "Paw Patrol" or "Peppa the Pig" and forget the mask is on. Children also do really well with charts and prizes. Every night your child wears the mask, reward them with a sticker of their choice on a visual poster board. Overtime, stickers could add up to "prizes" or special outings. You will be amazed how these little humans take to positive airway pressure therapy overtime (sometimes even better than adults!)

Also, to note, don't forget to use the RAMP feature on the CPAP machine to allow your child to fall asleep comfortably.

Conclusion

Thank you for reading this book!

I hope this book was able to help you learn about sleep apnea and the various treatment options for it. Also, I hope you were able to learn the pros and cons of each treatment to help you make a more informed and educated decision when it comes to your own treatment plan.

The next step is to make sure you consult a physician, respiratory therapist, or sleep team to see which treatments work best for you. Above all else, make sure to ask lots of questions, and make sure you understand what you are being treated for.

After all, it is your health! I sincerely hope you found value here. If there is even one or two bits that you can use going forward, then my job is done.

One more thing: I'd like to ask you for a favor. Would you be kind enough to leave a review for this book? It would be greatly appreciated. It's really quick at this link:

Click Here or copy this link:
https://www.amazon.com/review/create-review?&asin=B01BU9U6OE#

I am very open to feedback. If you think there is anything we can improve here, email me at info@resplabs.com

Thank you and good luck!

Brady

Brady Nelson RRT

Appendix 1 – Cleaning Your CPAP

For CPAP <u>Tube</u> Cleaning: Type **"CPAP Brush"** on YouTube.

For CPAP <u>Mask</u> Cleaning: Type "CPAP Wipes" on YouTube.

Your CPAP machine must be cleaned to keep it in good working order. When you're issued the machine, you're warned to use only distilled water in it. That's not because distilled water is somehow sterile; it's not. Distilled water, however, doesn't have minerals in it that can leave deposits behind in your machine. You might think, "Hey, as long as I use that and not tap water, I'm good to go, right?" But if you don't clean your CPAP machine, bacteria can build up inside that can eventually make you sick. Fortunately, cleaning the machine is actually pretty simple.

There's one thing you have to understand before we start, and that is that you're not actually cleaning the CPAP machine itself. You know, the gadget you actually plug in, with the electronic display and whatnot? You shouldn't ever put that in water or wipe it down with water. It's all the things plugged into the CPAP machine that you need to clean. These are...

- [ ] The mask
- [ ] The hose/tubing
- [ ] The humidifier chambers
- [ ] The filter(s) on the machine (which you're not cleaning, but replacing)

The first thing you'll want to do is buy yourself a little basin to wash your CPAP gear in. You can get these at your local drug store and even your local dollar store. It's just a plastic bucket that's lower and wider than an actual bucket. You know, it's the size of something you'd soak your feet in. The reason you want to buy one rather than use something you already have is that you should use this basin ONLY for your CPAP machine. You don't want to wash the CPAP gear in your sink unless you keep your sink spotlessly clean, and then only in the bathroom sink, not the kitchen. (Kitchen sinks tend to accumulate food particles and bacteria.)

Personally, I have no faith that I can get my bathroom sink clean enough that I'd want to basically breathe out of it, so when it comes to a CPAP machine, only clean its components in the basin you bought specifically for that purpose. You want to wash your CPAP machine in warm, soapy water. Don't use anything else. You don't want a harsh chemical soap, or anything like that. You just want something mild you can use to clean the components. Never use bleach or any other heavy chemical cleaner.

To clean the mask and tubing, take everything apart. Don't soak your headgear; there's no need to do that. Headgear eventually gets nasty from contact with your skin, which is why your insurance company will typically make provision to replace it periodically. Padding the headgear with a bandanna, between the straps and your scalp, will help it to last longer and prevent it from irritating your skin. You can also get soft strap pads to prevent red marks and further irritation.

For longest mask life, you can wash your face before you go to bed at night, to slow the gradual breakdown of the rubbery material that makes up the mask seal. Some people do clean the headgear but dipping it in water will leave it wet for much longer. Don't put your headgear in the washer or dryer, as it won't survive the trip. Masks, headgear, and cushions are designed to be replaced periodically, so know the recommended schedule and decide to buy the replacements. If your CPAP is subsidized by insurance, you'll be made aware, periodically, of the replacement schedule.

Remember, you're going to need to allow time for the mask and tubing to air-dry. I soak everything in the basin after filling it with warm water and mild soap, then place everything on folded paper towels to dry. This is best done in the early afternoon, say, after you get home from work at the latest, so that everything will be reasonably dry by evening. If you can do it in the morning, so much the better, as it will have that much longer to air-dry. Never put your equipment in direct sunlight, such as in a ray of sunshine from the bathroom or kitchen window because

UV radiation is bad for the material used in the mask and tube.

The humidifier chamber, which actually holds the distilled water, is where calcification and bacteria will tend to build up most over time. The chamber is designed to be taken apart, so you can clean it. Do so, and wipe it down with a warm, wet cloth. For a deeper clean once a week, you can soak it for twenty minutes in a solution of white vinegar and water (one parts vinegar to three parts water). Some manufacturers stipulate that their humidifiers are dishwasher safe, but honestly, the idea of putting my humidifier chamber in my dishwasher is just gross. If you do, only wash the chamber by itself, with no other dishes or any food particles, and make sure the dishwasher is completely clean before you run the cycle. Don't use the heat-drying feature, either. The last thing you want to do is bake food particles onto your humidifier.

Change your CPAP filters per the recommended schedule provided by your CPAP manufacturer, as advised by your sleep clinic doctor. The white, paper-like filters are disposable in most cases, so you don't need to worry about cleaning them, just changing them out. There may also be a gray, non-disposable filter on the back of your CPAP that can be rinsed or wiped down at least weekly. If you keep a very clean house, you won't notice much debris on the filter, but if you have pets, or lots of dust in your house, the filter will get dirty faster.

There are some cleaning products on the market that can make the task of cleaning your CPAP machine a little easier. These include, but are not limited to...

CPAP Brushes: You can buy CPAP tube brushes that are specially designed for scrubbing the inside of the CPAP tubing. It's designed like a plumbing snake, with a long flexible handle and a brush on the other end. Just run it through the tube, back and forth, to scrub the walls of the tubing gently. Remember, don't be too aggressive. Let the brush do the work for you so you don't damage the tubing. Most machines will use the standard width brushes, but some machines have slim tubing that require a smaller sized brush. Save yourself the time and purchase a CPAP brush that has the capacity to clean all CPAP tubing. If you are interested, learn more at our resource list at **RespLabs.com.**

CPAP Mask Wipes: Mask wipes are available that look a lot like the antibacterial wipes you buy to clean your hands, or the furniture polish wipes you buy for use on wood and countertops. You take the wipes and clean out the inside of the mask. The wipes make it much easier to remove debris, skin grease, and other residues that build up on the mask. Remember, you must use CPAP wipes, never anything with alcohol-based cleaning solution in it. Alcohol, just like bleach, ultraviolet radiation, or other harsh chemicals, will break down the material used to form the mask seal. If you are interested, learn more at our resource list at **RespLabs.com.**

So Clean 2: This is an automated CPAP cleaner that you use much like a dishwasher for your mask and tubing. There's no water, no chemicals, and no need to take things apart or dip them in water. You just put the mask and tubing inside the So Clean while it's connected to the

CPAP machine. The machine does the rest, sanitizing the water in the humidifier, the walls of the humidifier chamber, the hose, and the mask, all with a molecule called ozone (O3). The machine is roughly $200-300, makes cleaning a breeze, which makes it much easier to keep your machine nice and clean. The whole cycle works in about fifteen minutes (although the CPAP machine should be allowed to "rest" for two hours afterward). If you are interested, learn more at our resource list at **RespLabs.com.**

So Clean Travel CPAP Cleaner: This is a more compact version of the So Clean unit that is designed to be taken with you when you travel. Instead of placing the mask inside the machine, you put the mask inside a bag that serves the same purpose. If you are interested, learn more at our resource list at **RespLabs.com.**

Lumin CPAP Cleaner: The Lumin is a UV light CPAP cleaner that was launched on 2018. It appears that you basically slide your mask and or accessories into a drawer with mirrors and a UV light. At first glance, it seems like a great idea. UV light is used as a cleaner in hospitals frequently. I'm not sure the light would penetrate the deeper crevasses of a cpap mask that you would get with an ozone cleaner like the soclean. I see this as a potential drawback. If you are interested, learn more at our resource list at **RespLabs.com.**

Hurricane Drier: You can use the Hurricane Drier to eliminate moisture that builds up during cleaning, or when using the heated humidifier (sometimes water builds up in the tubing through normal use). It uses gentle, static air to dry your CPAP and CPAP accessories.

Do you need elaborate machinery to clean and sanitize your CPAP? Strictly speaking, no, because you can wash it manually and then let it air-dry. Machines like the So Clean and Hurricane Drier make it easier and simpler to conduct your regular cleaning, though. Which are you more likely to do? — drag out a basin, soap, and water, and scrub your tubing with a brush... or simply hook the mask up to a machine, press a button, and come back later?

However you choose to do it, however much money you spend on cleaning supplies, take the time to clean your CPAP machine on a regular basis. For best results, make it a part of your weekly routine, such as on a Sunday when you're thinking about the coming week. Proper cleaning of your CPAP machine will ensure the longest life for the machine and accessories, while preventing any unnecessary problems associated with the buildup of bacteria or other debris.

Appendix II - Respiratory Therapy

I can't finish this book without a quick word about our profession. I've had the privilege of working with thousands of patients and incredible colleagues as a respiratory therapist, which I'm very proud of.

For those that don't know what a respiratory therapist is, we are allied health professionals that manage patient's breathing in the community and for acute care. A typical day can range from asthma or sleep apnea education in the community, to managing the most traumatic patient's ventilation in the ER. I have many colleagues who practice all over the world who also love their profession.

If you know someone who would fit a role like this, I'd encourage you to talk to him or her about it and do some more research. There are plenty of schools across North America. The profession is growing globally.

If you have any questions about respiratory therapy, you can always email me at info@resplabs.com. Just write

Question for Brady in the subject line so it will be properly routed to me.

About the Author:

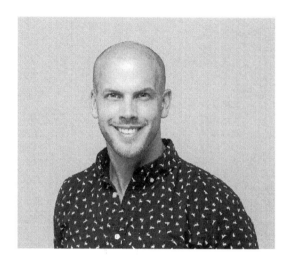

BRADY NELSON RRT, Brady is a Registered Respiratory Therapist with Experience in Acute & Community Care, as well as the Medical Device Industry. As a Director of RespLabs Medical Inc. he plays a key role as a provider of solutions that Make CPAP Simple (Continuous Positive Airway Pressure) for those with Sleep Apnea. Cleaning, Comfort, Filtration and other solutions to name a few.

He is also Co-Founder of RespiratoryExam.com, a Practice-Exam Platform for Respiratory Therapy Students to Prepare for Mid-terms, Finals & Licensing Exams.

More at **RespLabs.com**

Recommendation:

If you want to hear first hand from a patient who went through the ringer and back, look no further than Phil Elmore.

Phil's book: "10 Things Doctors Won't Tell You About Sleep Apnea", is short, to the point, frankly, made me laugh out loud a few times. (Not at his condition, the guy has a great sense of humor). His first-hand experience is likely shared by millions of other Sleep apnea sufferers. The way he laid it out in his book will resonate with you and the tips will be well worth it.

Click Here to Learn More: Amazon.com/Things-Doctors-Wont-About-Machine-ebook/dp/B015YHVOFI/

References:

1. American Thoracic Society. (2009, February 9). Losing Weight Can Cure Obstructive Sleep Apnea In Overweight Patients, Study Shows. Science Daily. Retrieved February 6, 2016 from www.sciencedaily.com/releases/2009/02/0902060 81319.htm

2. Lin YN, Li QY, Zhang XJ. Interaction between smoking and obstructive sleep apnea: Not just participants. Chin Med J (Engl) 2012;125:3150–6.

3. Kátia C. Guimarães, Luciano F. Drager, Pedro R. Genta, Bianca F. Marcondes, and Geraldo Lorenzi-Filho "Effects of Oropharyngeal Exercises on Patients with Moderate Obstructive Sleep Apnea Syndrome", American Journal of Respiratory and Critical Care Medicine, Vol. 179, No. 10(2009), pp. 962-966. doi: 10.1164/rccm.200806-981OC

4. Ieto V, Kayamori F, Montes MI, Hirata RP, Gregório MG, Alencar AM, Drager LF, Genta PR, Lorenzi-Filho G. Effects of Oropharyngeal Exercises on Snoring: A Randomized Trial. Chest. 2015 Sep;148(3):683-91. doi: 10.1378/chest.14-2953.

5. Puhan, M. A., Suarez, A., Lo Cascio, C., Zahn, A., Heitz, M., & Braendli, O. (2006). Didgeridoo

playing as alternative treatment for obstructive sleep apnoea syndrome: randomised controlled trial. *BMJ : British Medical Journal,332*(7536), 266–270. http://doi.org/10.1136/bmj.38705.470590.55

6. Positional therapy for obstructive sleep apnea: An objective measurement of patients' usage and efficacy at home. Heinzer, Raphael C. et al. Sleep Medicine , Volume 13 , Issue 4 , 425 – 428

7. Vorona RD; Ware JC; Sinacori JT; Ford ML; Cross JP. Treatment of severe obstructive sleep apnea syndrome with a chinstrap. *J Clin Sleep Med 2007*;3(7):729–730. http://www.ncbi.nlm.nih.gov/pmc/articles/PMC2 556917/

8. Sushanth Bhat, Neola Gushway-Henry, Peter G. Polos, Vincent A. DeBari, Sandeep Riar, Divya Gupta, Liudmila Lysenko, Disha Patel, Justin Pi, Sudhansu ChokrovertyJ Clin Sleep Med. 2014 August 15; 10(8): 887–892. Published online 2014 August 15. doi: 10.5664/jcsm.3962 http://www.ncbi.nlm.nih.gov/pmc/articles/PMC4 106943/

9. Effect of nasal-valve dilation on obstructive sleep apnea. B. Schönhofer, K. A. Franklin, H. Brünig, H. Wehde, D. Köhler Chest. 2000 September; 118(3): 587–590. http://www.ncbi.nlm.nih.gov/pubmed/10988176

10. Soose RJ, Woodson BT, Gillespie MB, Maurer JT, de Vries N, Steward DL, Strohl KP, Baskin JZ, Padhya TA, Badr MS, Lin HS, Vanderveken OM, Mickelson S, Chasens E, Strollo PJ Jr; STAR Trial Investigators. Upper Airway Stimulation for Obstructive Sleep Apnea: Self-reported Outcomes at 24 Months. J Clin Sleep Med. 2015 Jul 24. pii: jc-00477-14. [Epub ahead of print] http://www.ncbi.nlm.nih.gov/pubmed/26235158

11. Irshaad O. Ebrahim, olin M. Shapir, Adrian J. Williams, Peter B. Fenwick. Alcohol and Sleep: Effects on normal sleep. 24 January 2013: Alcoholism JournalVolume 37, Issue April 2013 Pages 539`–549. https//onlinelibrary.wiley.com/doi/10.1111/acer.1 2006/full

12. Open Anesthesia. Airway Pediatric vs Adult. Miller R. Pediatric anesthesia. Miller's Anesthesia. 6th ed. 2005. Elsevier, Churchill, Livingston. pp. 2384-8https://www.openanesthesia.org/airway_pediatri c_vs_adult/

Hacking CPAP Comfort

100+ Incredible Tips from Experts & Experienced Users.

This section of the book was made just for **CPAP users.**

It has been compiled and filtered from 7 Registered Respiratory Therapists who've treated thousands of patients, and over 100 experienced individual CPAP users.

The hardest part about putting this guide together, was deciding what information needs to be **left out**, so we could keep it to the most important points **only**. We've Hacked CPAP comfort down into a list of **100+** all around comfort hacks and tips.

If you have **just** been prescribed CPAP, this is definitely for you too.

If you've been CPAP for a **decade or more**, I guarantee there are still tips that will make your life easier.

I want to arm you with the power to minimize, decrease or fully remove any discomfort you are feeling using CPAP...FAST

No more fluff. Let's get to it...

The Most Important Factor in Comfort — Mask Fit

A proper mask fit is **the most** vital part of CPAP therapy. If there is anything to spend more money on, it is the mask.

Seriously. If you need to spend less on a machine to get a mask that fits best for you, do it. This isn't saying to buy the most expensive mask. Buy the mask that you think is the **most comfortable** and **leak-free**. You might be surprised, and since every face is different, there is no one-size-fits-all.

To get mask fitting **right**, we have to recommend a visit to a sleep clinic where you can trial **more than one** type. It will contribute to your success. At least for the 1st mask you get.

PS: Make sure to buy your mask from the sleep clinic that fits you, their service is highly worth it.

i.e. Don't buy your first mask online.

The 100+ CPAP Comfort Hacks

1) In each mask, there is an **intentional leak** to allow you to exhale through, as the CPAP system only has one tube to inhale and exhale from. This is called an exhalation port. It is important to make sure that this is leaking at all times, although, the mask should not be leaking in your eyes or under your nose. Make sure you ask your clinician where the intentional leak from the mask is coming from, as each mask is different. This leak will prevent you from re-breathing exhaled air, which can be dangerous.

2) A properly fit mask will not leave marks on your face for **more than an hour**. Make sure your straps are not too tight as this can not only lead to pressure sores but further leaking. It will depend on age and skin elasticity, how fast it returns to normal. Below are solutions to specific facial mark and pressure sore issues.

3) For facial marks related to your **headgear** you can use CPAP Strap Covers: **RespLabs.com.** They are very soft and will disperse the pressure exerted on your face (therefore reducing the marks). You can also seek a mask that has wider headgear straps, as the wider the straps, the more pressure distribution, the lesser the strap marks.

4) For facial marks related to your **mask** you can get CPAP Mask Liners: **RespLabs.com.** There are reusable and single-use versions. Mask liners protect your skin from the irritation. If you experience chaffing or acne from your mask, mask liners can help with that.

5) For **Neck** irritation, you can use a CPAP Neck Pad. They are soft to the touch and will disperse the pressure exerted on your neck. Get one here: **RespLabs.com**

6) For **forehead** marks related to your mask, there are CPAP gel pads for this problem.

7) For marks on the **bridge** of your nose, both Gel Pads or CPAP Mask Liners that can disperse the pressure over your nose and help prevent pressure sores in this area.

8) For **Pressure Sores**, you must treat them fast, or they will only get worse. Sometimes it means you need to just leave them alone. If you can use another CPAP mask that doesn't touch this area until it heals, that would be most optimal. A simple bandage over the affected area can work. A product used in the hospital for this purpose is called Duoderm. You may also switch from one style of mask to another for a night until heals.

9) Sometimes a simple **waterproof** bandage over the problem spot may help.

10) Duoderm is a really good **"second skin"** that we've used with patients in the hospital that had pressure sores from their CPAP masks. Use it to cover the sore when the CPAP mask is on, but make sure to not pull the mask on too tight on subsequent nights. You can get this product from a well-stocked drug store.

11) If you cannot solve the problem by simple adjustments of the mask and headgear, you may need to get a different mask that better fits you for the **long term**.

12) It is **normal** to have some marks in the morning (just as you would have if you slept on a crease of the sheets). At first sight after removing your mask the marks will be at their worst, but the majority of them will diminish fairly quickly, depending on your age and skin's elasticity.

13) Rub your skin with your fingers in **circular movements** to increase the blood flow and stretch the marked skin.

14) Use skin **concealers** and foundation, but choose powder-based ones, as liquid ones can get into the creases and make the marks look worse.

Mask Leak?

15) If you feel like you are **not** getting enough air, first be sure that you have turned on the machine. A small amount of air does come out while the machine is warming up, but you need to turn the pressure on to get enough air. If the machine is on, you may have a mask leak that is letting most of the air escape. If this is the case, you can adjust the mask as your clinician has recommended or replace it.

16) If your mask leaks in your eyes from time to time and you suffer from dry eyes, try wearing an eye mask to bed. Not only will it help you sleep by darkening your sight, but also will help with protection of your eyes. (if not an eye-mask, use a low-profile **tanning** bed mask)

17) Do not block the exhalation port between the mask and the connecting tubing from the device as this leak is your exhalation port. Position the port **away** from your bed partner as this leaking has sometimes known to annoy bed partners.

Mask Liners

18) Mask Liners are great for anyone feeling uncomfortable where their mask rests on their face, providing an **additional** barrier for comfort too.

19) Mask liners protect your skin from the **irritating** silicone. If you experience chaffing or acne from your mask, mask liners can help.

20) Mask liners also reduce noisy air leaks and protect your skin from **excessive** moisture. The reduction in moisture reduces skin irritation and mask leaks.

21) The liner material also prevents the cushion from slipping and **absorbing** facial oils which tend to loosen the mask seal.

22) Mask Liners are available in **Single-Use** or **Reusable**, washable options.

Headgear Hacks:

23) In order to fit your mask, the same every time, take your headgear off by un-velcroing **ONE** side only.

24) Draw a line with a **sharpie** felt on your headgear to indicate where to pull the fabric through to. This will help prevent over tightening.

25) Always secure the lower straps **before** securing the upper straps, this will prevent over tightening the upper strap and causing pressure sores on the bridge of the nose (most common).

26) When putting on your headgear, make sure to pull the two sides of the headgear at the **same** time. This will help keep the mask centered on your face and prevent leaking.

27) If your headgear has narrow or **irritating** straps, invest in CPAP strap covers.

28) CPAP strap covers are usually wider than the headgear and more comfortable (made with fleece usually) and have been shown to help with red marks in the morning by distributing the pressure **over a larger area**. Here they are again: **RespLabs.com.**

29) Headgear becoming loose after repetitive use may cause a leak. Just run it under the tap with warm water for about 1 minute. Squeeze out water and leave to dry. This can return the headgear to its **original form**.

30) Most headgear options secure around the base of your neck. This can be irritating for patients as sometimes the material the headgear is made of will leave people itchy and irritates the skin. See the Original **CPAP Neck Pad** here: **RespLabs.com**

Bloating? (Aerophagia or gas in stomach)

31) Bloating can be a sign you are **swallowing** the CPAP air. There is no real medical solution, but we have found that your sleeping position may be a factor.

32) First, try sleeping as flat as possible, even **without** a pillow. If the bloating persists, try sleeping on your side or elevated.

33) Try to avoid swallowing air. If you're new to CPAP, you may be swallowing air rather than breathing normally, which can cause bloating. When using your therapy device, breathe as normally as possible.

Facial Hair?

The biggest impact your facial hair has on your CPAP therapy is reducing the effectiveness of the seal for your CPAP treatment. Facial hair creates a barrier between your mask and your skin, which leads to increased mask leaks. This results in your CPAP therapy being less effective and your sleep apnea not being treated as effectively.

34) Consider shaving **or** trimming your facial hair. Completely shaving your facial hair will be most effective in improving your current mask seal but trimming down the thickness of your beard or mustache can help as well.

If You Have Tried Everything…

35) If your mask isn't fitting right (leaking at night or causing skin irritation and pressure sores) first, try refitting the mask as your **clinician** has recommended.

36) Try a different **size** mask. If you can only get a good seal by tightening the mask until it's uncomfortable, then you may have the wrong size.

Humidification...

The reason that most CPAP machines come with a humidifier is because the pressurized air you are breathing is coming in a lot faster than room air. Our noses are our body's mini "humidifier". The nose has three jobs: to filter, heat and humidify the air we breathe. When the air passes so quickly from the CPAP machine to our lungs, the nose has to work overtime to do its job.

There are different types of humidifiers in CPAP machines. One is a pass-over humidifier. This works passively and is not heated. The air passes over water, picking up water droplets before it makes its way to your mask. The other is a heated humidifier, a heated water pot that adds heated water to the tubing, and therefore to you.

Using a Humidifier:

37) A CPAP heated humidifier can **prevent a dry mouth** and **sinus problems** caused by the stream of pressurized air.

38) A CPAP heated humidifier works by using a fine mist of warm or room-temperature distilled water to keep your **nasal passages moist.**

39) Ask your clinician to go over the operation of the humidifier with you in detail. Generally, the humidifiers range in scale from 1 to 5. The "lowest" setting is 1 and therefore, heats the water the least and results in less water output from the humidifier, leaving you feeling dry. The higher you place the humidifier setting on, the higher the **humidity output**, and therefore the more humidified the air you breathe. In our experience, most patients find a setting in the middle the most comfortable (3-4).

40) Remember that the temperature of the **room** can affect the humidity output and the amount of condensation in the tubing as well. The colder the room, generally the more rain-out.

Using Distilled Water:

41) Use **distilled** water only to fill your humidifier as it helps prevent mold and mineral deposit build up in your humidifier base.

42) Distilled water is the purest water and is recommended for the CPAP humidifier use to keep your machine **hygienic** and operating properly.

Heated Tubing Tips:

43) Heated tubing can help prevent "rain-out" or condensation in the tubing caused by air cooling from the **humidifier** to the **mask**. Sometimes, condensation can get really bad and cause pooling of water in the tubing and your mask, leading to night time wake-ups.

44) Heated tubing helps with this as it heats the pressurized air all the way from the humidifier to the mask, **preventing** the process of condensation.

CPAP Hose Covers:

45) CPAP hose covers in **conjunction** with heated tubing can greatly reduce the amount of condensation in your tubing, and therefore your mask.

46) Pick a CPAP hose cover that feels good on your **skin** as you will most likely contact this material in the night.

47) For a soft and super comfortable, washable, fleece CPAP hose cover, find The Original RespLabs CPAP

Hose Cover in every size in our resource list at **RespLabs.com**

The Location of Your CPAP Machine is Important!

48) Place your CPAP machine **2 feet** under the height of your mattress. Gravity will prevent condensation from your CPAP machine entering your mask.

49) A neat trick to help with better rain out drainage is to use an old tie over the bed post. Thread the CPAP tube through the tie and down to the mattress. This results in no more **drag** on the mask and better rain out drainage. A CPAP hose clip can also help you with this here: **RespLabs.com**

Staying Hydrated:

50) A practical tip is to keep a bottle of water by your bed or a cup with a lid but only drink **just enough** water to wet your mouth, as drinking can cause you to inhale any liquid (or food) if taken too close to your sleep time and can aggravate acid reflux.

51) Use a **straw** to drink from as it will be easier with the mask on your face.

52) Increase your level of comfort by using a **saline** spray as a nasal moisturizer.

Moisturize, Moisturize, Moisturize...

53) Another common problem a CPAP user experiences is skin irritation, such as dryness, cracking, and chafing, from the use of their CPAP mask. Use a CPAP moisture therapy cream and apply it to affected areas as often as needed.

54) Petroleum-based products should **<u>not</u>** be used with CPAP masks since most are made of silicone. Petroleum may break down the silicone on CPAP masks causing damage and therefore, shorten the lifespan of the mask. Petroleum-based products (like vaseline) are unsafe with the use of CPAP machines, especially those with oxygen tee'd into them.

55) RespLabs Medical's CPAP lotion, CPAP Chap, was made for patients on CPAP to help prevent and soothe skin irritation from CPAP use. It is **petroleum-free**, completely safe for CPAP users. Plus, it is packed with vitamin E which restores moisture and blocks free radicals and vitamin A & Aloe Vera to heal damaged skin and reduce inflammation. Visit our resource list to learn more at **RespLabs.com**.

Getting Accustomed:

56) The biggest thing about CPAP is to learn to accept its presence and be patient to stick with it. The reality is that the **less** you wear the mask, the harder it will be to get used to wearing it. It will take some time before you are fully accustomed to the feeling of wearing the mask in bed. CPAP is not a quick fix for your problem. It involves commitment to improve your sleep and health.

57) Give yourself time to get used to therapy. Acknowledge the effort that you made and commit to having a better night the next evening. Give yourself at least **6 weeks'** time to trial the CPAP machine. If you give yourself this time, you can work out any kinks. There **will** be kinks along the way.

Wearing the Mask When Awake:

58) Hold the mask to your face **without** it strapped on. Turn on your CPAP machine for 10 minutes and hold the mask in place while awake and watching TV.

59) If you have a **RAMP** option, your CPAP pressure will start lower and then ramp up until the prescribed pressure is reached. For example, if you are prescribed a CPAP pressure of 10 cmH20, and you choose the RAMP option, the machine will take some time to build pressure and may start as low as 4 cmH20. Press the RAMP button and allow yourself some time to breathe with the lower pressure to get used to the feeling. Over the course of 10-30 minutes, the CPAP machine will ramp up the pressure to the prescribed level.

Most new CPAP users find the feeling of the pressurized air on their face very uncomfortable. It can feel like holding your head out of a car window. In order to be able to fall asleep with the CPAP machine on, this is where the RAMP options can really help.

60) You can wear the mask **while** watching television or reading. The activity will distract you, while you get more accustomed to the feeling and any weight of the mask. **NEVER** attach yourself to the machine without turning the flow of gas ON as this can lead to rebreathing exhaled gas.

Sleep Log:

61) The use of a **sleep log** may help you focus on which of the insomnia triggers are most critical to address and solve, and those which can wait. It may also help you see subtle, but positive changes in how you are feeling with the use of CPAP. Keeping a sleep log is not all that difficult. You can use a notebook or a spreadsheet to do it.

Every MORNING after you get up write down the following information:

- What time you actually went to bed
- Estimate of how long it took you to fall asleep
- Estimate of how many times you woke up during the night
- Time you got up for the morning
- Estimate of total time you slept during the night
- Comments on how you feel upon waking up for the day
- Additional comments on any wakes that you feel were disruptive or problems you had getting to sleep

There are apps now that make this easier.

Don't Fight It:

Lying in bed for hours while awake and fighting with the mask is counterproductive. It's teaching your body how to stay awake and resist the mask instead of sleeping with the mask

62) Allow yourself to spend about **30** minutes fighting the leaks or the mask straps or the feeling that you cannot stand to have the mask on your face. But at the end of 30 minutes, if you are not sleepy and still actively fighting with the mask, get out of bed, go into a different room and do something that will help you get your mind off the mask.

Sleep Hygiene Tips:

Make sure that you're practicing good sleep hygiene. Sleep hygiene consists of practices, rituals, and choices that help you get to sleep on time, stay asleep longer, and have restorative sleep every night. If you develop healthy sleep habits and good sleep hygiene, you will take to CPAP easier and faster than those who don't.

63) Exercise **regularly** and avoid caffeine and alcohol before bedtime.

64) Eliminate **non-essential** electronics (cell phones, TVs) from the bedroom.

65) Decide on a nightly bedtime **routine** to get your mind and body ready for sleep

66) Keep a **consistent** schedule for **going to bed** and **waking up**.

67) Perform **relaxation** exercises to assist with sleep. Learn more by typing "relaxation exercises" on YouTube.

68) Improve your **sleeping environment** by purchasing a good mattress and pillow and making sure your bedroom is dark, quiet and the right temperature. It is recommended that your bedroom's temperature is between 16 and 20 degrees Celsius. If you can't control the noise or light of you room, invest in ear plugs and eye masks.

69) If you like your room darkened (most people do), Use **black-out** blinds.

70) Don't go to bed **until** you feel tired. If you head off to bed when you aren't feeling tired, you may not be able to switch off. Add in the addition of something new and unfamiliar like a CPAP machine, and you might find it unusually hard to fall asleep.

71) Avoid stressful, stimulating activities like doing work or discussing emotional issues. These kinds of activities can cause the body to **secrete** the stress hormone cortisol, which is associated with increasing alertness.

Breathing your way to sleep.

72) You can **breathe your way to sleep** through your CPAP machine. Find a comfortable position in bed. Let yourself relax and start to notice your body and any sensations you feel. Feel the connection between your body and the surface you're lying on. Relax any tension and soften your muscles. Start to notice your breath and where you feel it in your body. You might feel it in your abdomen, your chest, or in your nostrils. Focus your attention on the full breath, from **start to finish.** If your mind is wandering, just notice that it has wandered and gently redirect it back to your breath.

73) Take a deep breath into your **lower belly** (not your chest) and feel your abdomen expand with air. Hold this for a few seconds and then release. Notice your belly rising and falling, and the air coming in and out a few times. Imagine the air filling up your abdomen, and then traveling out your airways, over and over. Continue to do this for a few minutes, focusing your mind back to your body and the breath coming in and out. Any time a thought crosses your mind, release that thought and refocus on the breath.

Minimizing Noise

74) Minimizing noise will help you sleep at night. Most modern CPAP machines and masks are designed to be **more and more silent**. If your device is too noisy, check that is it set up correctly, the filter is   clean, and the machine air-intake is unobstructed. If these things are all checked and working well, try wearing earplugs or masking the sound of the machine with relaxing ambient noise. You can also always use the CPAP hose cover to diminish the sound amplification in your CPAP tubing. Check out the original CPAP Hose Cover in the resource list at **RespLabs.com**.

Aromatherapy:

75) Essential oils can be enjoyed right from a CPAP machine. Enjoy the fragrance of lavender, or the sweet scent of cherry or oranges. These may help in calming your **anxiety** while using CPAP during night time. Pleasant smells induce strong feelings of calm, comfort, and relaxation. The sense of smell is part of the brain's emotional centers and cognitive distraction (the ability to exclude other distracting stimuli).

76) Some people tend to feel claustrophobic when using their CPAP. Having relaxing scents delivered through the machine can reduce the anxiety levels to reach a higher comfort level. Use your favorite essential oils applied to a diffuser pad and placed **in front** of the machine's air intake port. (Not on the actual filter inside the air-intake).

However, a CPAP filter can easily be used as a diffuser pad, but it **must not** be used again as a CPAP air filter

NOTE on Oils:

77) You should **NOT** apply essential oils directly to the machine filter, because it could not only break down the machine filter, but it will also add air resistance to the machine making it work much harder than needed.

78) You should also **NOT** add the essential oil to the humidifier chamber water, it can then potentially reach deep into your lungs when you are only supposed to use it as a scent for the receptors of smell.

Cleaning Your CPAP:

79) Keeping your CPAP mask, tubing and humidifier clean are essential to your comfort on CPAP. If you are negligent and do not properly clean and wipe down your mask, tubing and humidifier you will open yourself up to **infection** risks.

80) Cleaning your CPAP mask is really easy! Use **mask wipes daily** in combination with **soap and water every 1 to 1.5 weeks**. For soap, use a mild dish detergent with warm water. Be very careful to not use disinfectants. They may damage your mask and gradually break down the soft silicone, a lot faster. CPAP mask wipes are designed to clean your mask daily and are a safe option for your mask. Get the Original CPAP Mask Wipes on our resource list at **RespLabs.com.**

CPAP Hose Cleaning

81) Cleaning your CPAP hose is a bit tougher and can sometimes be cumbersome using different buckets etc.

Clinicians will usually recommend **soaking** the tubing in warm soapy water and then sterilizing it with a ⅓ white vinegar to water solution.

82) Many users are not sure if they have cleaned their tubing enough and are worried about what can be accumulating, and hopefully not "growing" inside. We've designed a CPAP Brush for every tube (universal or slim line) and mask orifice available. It is **[8 in 1]** and you can get it in out resource list at **RespLabs.com.**

83) Hang your hose to air dry for 12 hours. A good place to hang your CPAP tubing is over a **shower rail**.

Humidifier Cleaning:

84) Your humidifier should also be cleaned in a warm soapy water solution and then sterilized with a ⅓ white vinegar to water solution. You can use the brush included with the original CPAP Brush in our resource list at **RespLabs.com.**

Air Filtration:

85) Always change your filters as per recommended by your clinician, and more often as needed. It is recommended to inspect your filters daily for signs of discoloration.

Sometimes, the slightest change in air pollution can change the filters dramatically. Dirty filters can not only open you up to **infection** but can actually cause your CPAP machine to **malfunction**!

86) Pollution adversely effects CPAP filters. We recently had forest fires in our area, and many patients had to go from changing their filters bi-weekly to **daily**! For a full list of CPAP filters, visit our resource list at **RespLabs.com**.

CPAP Cleaning Machines:

87) There are many different CPAP cleaning devices on the market. A SoClean machine can sanitize and clean all CPAP equipment (mask, hose, reservoir) in an automated fashion. Using the SoClean device will save you time and energy. The company claims that the machine destroys 99.9% of all germs and bacteria. You **need** to wipe down the mask and parts prior to use of a SoClean sanitizer. To get a SoClean device, visit our resource list at **RespLabs.com.**

There are other cleaners now like the SoClean that use ozone, about half the size of a standard brick. You can place cpap tubing directly onto one end of it. However, there is question about the amount of ozone each produce and are the levels safe for the items that are being cleaned. I learned about this first hand when a company was presenting one of these devices (They look the exact same from multiple companies).

Travelling with CPAP:

Once you've started using your CPAP every night, you will want to take it everywhere with you. Many patients on CPAP fear travelling as they think they will be unable to take their machines. The truth is, it can be very easy to travel with CPAP! Here are some tips for you:

88) If your CPAP comes with a marine battery, make sure to ask the clinician how long it will last for. Many of the CPAP batteries are expensive. Try going to a local store that sells electronics or homeware supplies. You can get a battery which you can run your CPAP machine for **much less**. Make sure it is compatible with the voltage of your CPAP machine.

89) If you take a flight to your destination, you will need to take your CPAP machine in your carry-on luggage. To identify your CPAP machine, use a **medical device luggage tag** like the one at **RespLabs.com**.

90) The above luggage tag can help identify your equipment for easy check in at security points. TSA guidelines state that Respiratory Equipment (CPAP or BiPAP machines) are allowable as carry-on luggage and should **NOT** be counted towards your carry-on allowance because they are medical necessities.

91) You can bring **individually wrapped** CPAP travel wipes on your trip to make sure your CPAP equipment is clean, on the go. You may not have access to buckets and sinks like you do at home, so CPAP travel wipes will allow you to keep your equipment germ free! See our resource list at **RespLabs.com**.

92) Most modern CPAP machines are lightweight, portable, and come with a specific carrying case. There are specific lightweight travel CPAP machines that are even more convenient to bring. Check with your provider for the best ones on the market. If you travel a lot, it may be worth it to purchase a specific travel machine.

93) Make sure you have all the proper **adaptors** and plugs for **foreign** countries.

94) Bring extra supplies (just in case your CPAP hose becomes compromised with a hole or your mask cushion rips). For a good choice of hoses and travel supplies, visit our resource list at **RespLabs.com**.

95) Remember to make sure your CPAP machine humidifier is **EMPTY**. You do not want to destroy your CPAP machine with water spillage throughout the internal parts.

96) If you are flying overnight, make sure to look into the airline you are flying with and inquire about **power outlets** at your seat. Some CPAP machines come with car charger ports. The plane may have these type of power outlets as well.

CPAP Pillows:

97) A CPAP Pillow can aide in the comfort of wearing a CPAP machine at night. The pillows are designed to position your neck, so your airway is more likely to remain open during sleep. These pillows have **contoured cut outs** for side sleeping and allow room for the mask and hose apparatus of a CPAP machine. Studies have shown that these pillows may help with mild sleep apnea symptoms and increase the comfort of those using CPAP machines. A CPAP pillow allows you to sleep in different positions, where standard pillows **do not** adapt to the mask.

A standard pillow cannot only cause leaking from your mask it also allows your head to tilt back and be unsupported while sleeping. This can result in pain in the joints of your jaw that feels like an earache when you wake up. By using a pillow specifically designed to contour and support your CPAP hose and mask it will keep your head and neck in the proper position and help to alleviate this pain.

CPAP Hose Holders:

98) CPAP hose clips can hook to a bed sheet, pillow case, nightstand, headboard, blanket and almost any other contraption at your bedside. This helps keep your CPAP tube from tangling into a knot or pulling away from your mask and causing accidental disconnections in the middle of the night. Visit our resource list to get them at **RespLabs.com.**

4 More CPAP DIY Tips:

99) You can use a Ladies **fabric headband** for a chinstrap. Just make sure that the material is comfortable for you and the headband is large enough to fit under your chin and over your head.

100) Use the **Hat-trick** for CPAP. A baseball cap helps both the top and back straps of the CPAP mask stay on, particularly for people who are bald, (or going that way like myself). The hat adds space, helping to reduce facial strap marks. The bill of the cap can help "lock" the position of the CPAP mask-tubing, making the whole system more secure and lessening the likelihood of leaks AND if the cap is worn backwards, it will keep people off of their back, the worst sleeping position for those with sleep apnea.

101) Use **hair-clips** to support the mask in place by securing the headgear in your hair with hair clips.

102) If you are unable to curb dry eyes with an eye mask, try a narrow swim or tanning **goggles**.

Conclusion

If you start using your CPAP machine every time you take a nap or go to sleep at night, you will find it becomes easier and easier to sleep with the CPAP mask on. Keep in mind the benefits that await you; better sleep leads to improved concentration, mood and energy, in turn improving your overall health and well-being.

Tracking your CPAP use is important for your success with CPAP. You can track your CPAP use on your computer or phone – just like you would track your steps on a fitness tracker. Challenge yourself to use your CPAP a little more each night and track your progress online. The apps for the different CPAP machines will even help you set goals and provide words of encouragement.

There are likely CPAP support groups in your area, and even on Facebook. If not, you can even start a CPAP support group in your community.

Creating a community of CPAP users that understand the difficulty faced in treating their disorder can work wonders on helping uplift others that are struggling with similar issues. New patients can attend and get the extra help, guidance, and assurances they need to get motivated to continue therapy. Seasoned patients can help those struggling by offering advice, tips and tricks, and share their own stories about their struggles wearing CPAP.

Thank you for reading this book. We hope you learned something that can help you with your CPAP journey. Many trained respiratory therapists have contributed to this book to help patients like YOU become more comfortable on CPAP.

I sincerely hope you found value here if there is even one or two bits that you can use going forward, then my job is done.

One more thing: I'd like to ask you for a favor. Would you be kind enough to leave a review for this book? It would be greatly appreciated. It's really quick at this link:

Click Here or visit this link:
amazon.com/review/create-review?&asin=B01BU9U6OE#

I am very open to feedback. If you think there is anything we can improve here, email me at info@resplabs.com

Thank you and good luck!

Cheers,

Brady

Brady Nelson RRT

I'd like to credit those that helped with Hacking CPAP Comfort:

Alisha Nelson RRT
Sheri Walker RRT
Opninder Lindstrom RRT
Stephanie Belanger RRT
Sunny Gill RRT
Erissa Limketee RRT
Phil Elmore, Author of "10 Things Your Doctor Won't Tell You About Your CPAP Machine"
Fiona Visika Suanding

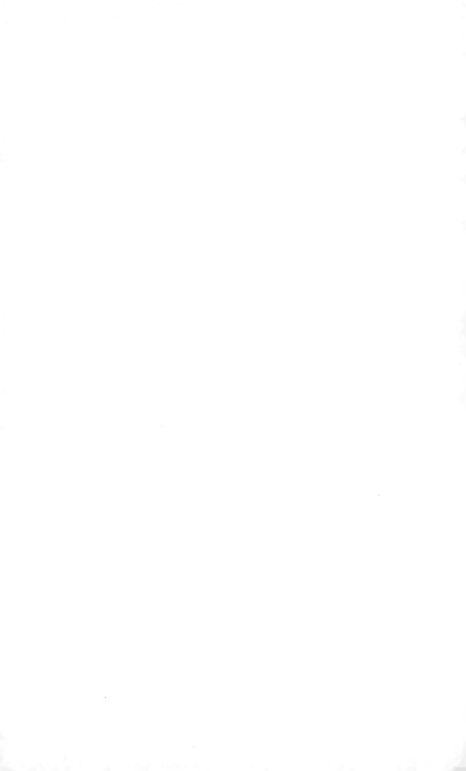

30328039R00082

Made in the USA
Middletown, DE
27 December 2018